How to Become a Veterinarian

A Complete Guide to Start a Career Working With Animals

Chris Hooper

Table of Contents

Chapter One

Veterinarian

Introduction

Understanding the veterinary profession

Understanding the veterinary profession involves understanding the multifaceted nature of the role and recognizing the responsibilities, challenges and rewards that come with it. Here are the key aspects to consider:

1. Passion for animals:

   - Deep and true love for animals is the foundation of the veterinary profession. This passion serves as a driving force behind efforts to improve the health and well-being of various species.

2. Different roles:

   -Veterinarians wear a variety of hats, from primary pet care providers to specialists in fields such as surgery, dentistry, pathology, and public health. Understanding the different roles within a profession helps individuals tailor their career path to their interests.

3. Lifelong learning:

   - The field of veterinary medicine is dynamic, with constant advances in technology,

treatment and research. Vets
must commit to lifelong learning
to keep up with new
developments and continually
improve their skills.

4. Communication skills:

 - Effective communication is
essential for veterinarians. They
need to convey comprehensive
medical information to pet
owners, collaborate with
colleagues, and educate the
public on animal health issues.
Strong interpersonal skills
contribute to successful outcomes
in veterinary practice.

5. Ability to solve problems:

- Veterinarians are often faced with diagnostic problems and unique cases. Developing strong problem-solving skills is essential for identifying and solving animal health problems, whether common or rare.

6. Ethical considerations:

- The veterinary profession involves navigating ethical dilemmas such as balancing the animal's best interests with the owner's wishes, weighing economic constraints, and making decisions in the face of uncertainty. A solid ethical framework is crucial.

7. Continuous professional development:

- Veterinary professionals engage in continuing education through conferences, workshops, and continuing education to stay abreast of medical advances. A commitment to professional development ensures that veterinarians provide the best possible care throughout their careers.

8. Teamwork:

- Veterinarians often collaborate with veterinary technicians, assistants and other professionals. Effective teamwork is essential for providing comprehensive care and managing the diverse challenges encountered in veterinary practice.

9. Emotional resilience:

   - The veterinary profession includes moments of joy as well as challenges, including difficult diagnoses, euthanasia decisions and emotional conversations with pet owners. Developing emotional resilience is essential to maintaining well-being and providing compassionate care.

10. Promotion of animal welfare:

- Veterinarians are animal welfare advocates, supporting responsible pet ownership, humane treatment of animals, and initiatives that contribute to the overall well-being of animals in society. This advocacy extends beyond clinical practice to broader community engagement.

11. Global Perspectives:

- Veterinary medicine is connected on a global scale. Veterinarians can contribute to international efforts such as disease control, wildlife conservation, and disaster response. A global perspective is valuable for addressing broader animal health issues.

12. Entrepreneurial spirit:

   - In addition to traditional roles, some vets may choose entrepreneurial paths such as owning their own practice or pursuing specialized specialties. An entrepreneurial mindset can lead to innovation and expansion of opportunities within a profession.

Understanding these aspects of the veterinary profession provides a foundation for individuals aspiring to enter the field and guides them through the challenges and embracing the fulfilling aspects of a career dedicated to animal welfare.

The importance of veterinarians in society

Veterinarians play a key role in society in a variety of areas, contributing to the health and well-being of animals, people and the environment. Here are some key aspects highlighting the importance of veterinarians in society:

1. Animal health and welfare:

   - Veterinarians are the main advocates of animal health and welfare. They diagnose and treat disease, prevent the spread of disease, and ensure that animals receive proper care, whether they are pets, farm animals, or wild animals.

2. Protection of public health:

   - By monitoring and controlling diseases that can be transmitted between animals and humans (zoonoses), veterinarians play a vital role in protecting public health. This includes disease surveillance, research and the implementation of preventive measures to reduce the risk of infectious diseases.

3. Food safety and security:

- Veterinarians contribute to the safety of the food chain by inspecting food production facilities, conducting research on foodborne pathogens, and implementing measures to prevent disease transmission through food products. Their efforts ensure that the food we consume is safe and free of contaminants.

4. One Health Initiatives:

- Veterinarians actively participate in One Health initiatives, recognizing the interconnectedness of human, animal and environmental health. Collaboration between veterinarians, health professionals, environmental scientists and other stakeholders leads to comprehensive solutions to global health problems.

5. Livestock production and agriculture:

- In the agricultural environment, veterinarians support the sustainability and productivity of livestock farming. They work to prevent and control disease, optimize herd health and ensure animal welfare. This contributes to the stability of food production systems and supports the livelihoods of farmers.

6. Disaster Response and Crisis
Management:

- Vets are critical to disaster
response and crisis management.
They play a key role in rescuing
and treating animals affected by
natural disasters such as fires or
hurricanes. Their expertise
ensures the well-being of
domestic and wild animals during
emergencies.

7. Preventive medicine and public
education:

- Vets emphasize preventive
medicine by promoting
vaccinations, wellness exams and
responsible pet ownership. They

also educate the public on issues such as parasite control, nutrition and behavior, which contribute to the overall health and happiness of pets and their owners.

8. Research and innovation:

- Veterinarians contribute to scientific research and innovation in areas such as veterinary medicine, animal behavior and pharmacy. Their work helps advance medical knowledge, leading to better treatments, diagnostic tools and technologies for both animals and humans.

9. Human-Animal Bond:

- Vets foster positive human-animal relationships and recognize the therapeutic benefits of the bond between people and their pets. Through preventive care and behavioral counseling, they increase the well-being and quality of life of animals and their owners.

10. Environmental protection:

- Vets play a role in wildlife conservation by addressing the health and well-being of endangered species. Their efforts contribute to the preservation of biodiversity and the balance of ecosystems.

Essentially, veterinarians are an integral part of the fabric of society and contribute to the health, safety and harmony of our interconnected world. Their diverse roles and expertise extend beyond the clinic to impact communities, agriculture, public health and the environment.

Overview of the path of veterinary education

The veterinary education pathway is a rigorous and comprehensive process that prepares individuals to become veterinarians. It usually involves several years of academic study, practical clinical experience and the development of basic skills. Here is an overview of the veterinary education path:

1. Pre-veterinary education (undergraduate studies):

   - Aspiring veterinarians typically begin their journey with a strong foundation in science. While specific requirements may vary, most veterinary schools expect applicants to complete a bachelor's degree with a concentration in pre-veterinary coursework. Common prerequisites include biology, chemistry, physics, mathematics, and sometimes additional courses in areas such as animal science or genetics.

2. Veterinary College Admission Test (VCAT):

   - Before applying to veterinary school, candidates are often required to take the Veterinary College Admission Test (VCAT). Similar to the Medical College Admission Test (MCAT) for medical school, the VCAT assesses a candidate's academic ability and scientific knowledge.

3. Application for veterinary school:

   - The veterinary school application process is highly

competitive. Applicants typically submit transcripts, letters of recommendation, a personal statement, and their VCAT scores. Some programs may also require interviews as part of the selection process.

4. Veterinary school (doctor of veterinary medicine - MVDr. Program):

   - Veterinary School is a four-year program leading to a Doctor of Veterinary Medicine (DVM) degree. The curriculum is intensive and covers a wide range of topics, including anatomy, physiology, pharmacology, pathology, surgery and clinical skills. Students spend the first two years of classroom instruction, followed by two years of clinical rotations where they gain hands-on experience working with patients.

5. Clinical rotations:

- Clinical rotations allow veterinary students to gain hands-on experience in a variety of specialty areas such as internal medicine, surgery, radiology, dermatology, and more. This hands-on training is key to developing clinical skills and decision-making abilities.

6. Licensing exams:

- After completing the DVM
program, graduates must pass
licensing exams to practice
veterinary medicine. In the
United States, this often involves
passing the North American
Veterinary Licensing Examination
(NAVLE). Each country may have
its own licensing requirements
and exams.

7. Internships and residencies
(optional):

- Some veterinarians choose to
receive additional training
through internships or
residencies, especially if they are
interested in specializing in a
particular field of veterinary

medicine. This can add a few more years to the education journey.

8. State license:

- Veterinarians must obtain a license to practice in a specific state or country. Licensing requirements vary, but usually include passing required exams and meeting other state-specific criteria.

9. Further education:

- The field of veterinary medicine is constantly evolving and veterinarians are required to engage in continuing education to stay current with advancements in the field. This may include attending conferences, workshops and other certifications.

The journey of veterinary education is challenging but rewarding, preparing individuals to provide high quality animal care and contribute to the wider field of veterinary medicine. It takes dedication, a passion for animal health and a commitment to lifelong learning.

Chapter Two

Discovering Your Passion

Embarking on the journey to becoming a veterinarian begins with a fundamental exploration of your passions in the diverse field of veterinary medicine. This serves as a guide to help you uncover your deepest interests and align them with the many opportunities the profession offers.

1. Examination of various veterinary specialties

Dive into the vast ocean of veterinary specialties, from small animal care to exotic species, wildlife conservation, surgery, pathology and more. Through anecdotes and insights from practicing veterinarians, gain a first-hand understanding of the different paths available in the field.

2. Gaining practical experience through volunteering and internships

Discovering your passion involves more than just theoretical knowledge. Engage in hands-on experience by volunteering at animal shelters, wildlife rehabilitation centers, or veterinary clinics. Internships provide valuable insights into day-to-day veterinary practice and allow you to witness the reality of different specialties.

3. Networking with veterinarians and veterinary professionals

Connect with seasoned professionals for valuable insights and advice. Attend veterinary conferences, seminars and workshops and interact with experts in various fields. Networking not only expands your understanding, but also opens the door to mentorship and potential opportunities in your field of interest.

4. Reflection of personal values
and goals

Consider your own values,
strengths, and long-term goals.
Think about how they align with
different aspects of veterinary
medicine. Whether your passion
lies in maintaining the human-
animal bond, contributing to
public health, or advocating for
wildlife conservation,
understanding your personal
aspirations is key to discovering
your unique path.

5. Seeking Mentorship

Mentors can provide invaluable
guidance as you navigate the

complexities of veterinary medicine. Find mentors in your areas of interest and ask them for advice. Learn from their experiences, challenges and triumphs and let their insights shape and refine your own aspirations.

6. Balancing passion and practicality

Passion is a driving force, but it needs to be balanced with practical considerations. Assess the requirements, lifestyle and potential challenges associated with your chosen path. Understanding the practical aspects will ensure that your

passion is aligned with a
sustainable and fulfilling career in
veterinary medicine.

7. Acceptance of Continuous
Survey

Passions can evolve as you
progress in your veterinary
education and career. Embark on
a journey of continuous
exploration and allow yourself the
flexibility to adapt and discover
new interests. The veterinary
profession offers a dynamic
landscape, and your passion can
take you to unexpected and
fulfilling destinations.

Building a Strong Educational Base

Establishing a solid educational foundation is a critical step on the path to becoming a veterinarian. This provides guidance on the essential components of your academic journey and ensures that you lay the foundations for a successful and fulfilling career in veterinary medicine.

1. Choosing the right high school courses

Begin your educational journey by choosing high school courses that align with veterinary school prerequisites. Focus on building a strong foundation in sciences such as biology, chemistry and physics. Math courses, especially algebra and statistics, will also add to your academic readiness.

2. Completion of a bachelor's degree in pre-veterinary studies

A common route to veterinary school is a bachelor's degree in pre-veterinary studies or a related field. Research college programs that offer a curriculum aligned with vet school prerequisites. Take advantage of opportunities to engage in research, extracurricular activities and leadership roles that will enrich your academic experience.

3. Understanding the courses necessary for veterinary school

Veterinary schools usually have specific courses that applicants must take. Familiarize yourself with these requirements, which often include biology, chemistry, physics, biochemistry, and mathematics. Make sure your undergraduate thesis is consistent with these prerequisites to strengthen your application to veterinary school.

4. Excelling in science and math courses

Mastering science and math courses is the foundation for

success in veterinary school. Develop effective study habits, seek additional support when needed, and actively participate in class discussions and lab work. A strong academic performance in these core courses will increase your overall competitiveness.

5. Participation in extracurricular activities and leadership roles

Involvement in extracurricular activities in addition to academics demonstrates a well-rounded and proactive approach. Join clubs, organizations, or volunteer programs related to animals, science, or community service. Seek leadership roles to demonstrate your initiative and ability to contribute to the team.

6. Building relationships with professors and mentors

Make meaningful connections with professors and mentors who can provide guidance and support. Attend office hours, participate in research projects, and seek mentorship from faculty members with expertise in veterinary medicine. These relationships can result in strong letters of recommendation for vet school applications.

7. Gaining Animal Experience and Exposure

Actively seek opportunities to gain hands-on experience with animals. Volunteer at animal shelters, farms, veterinary clinics or research facilities. This hands-on experience will not only strengthen your application, but also provide valuable insight into the day-to-day duties of a veterinarian.

8. Use of Research Opportunities

Get involved in research projects related to veterinary medicine or animal science. Research experience demonstrates your commitment to academic inquiry and contributes to your overall competitiveness when applying to veterinary school.

9. Exploring dual degree programs and specializations

Explore dual degree programs or specialized tracks offered by some universities. These programs can allow you to combine your veterinary studies with another field, such as public health or research, to provide a unique and enriching educational experience.

10. Maintaining a Strong GPA

Maintain a competitive grade point average (GPA) throughout your educational journey. A strong GPA is a critical factor in veterinary school admissions, reflecting your academic dedication and readiness for rigorous coursework.

Chapter Three

Preparing for the Veterinary College Entrance Examination (VCAT)

The Veterinary College Admission Test (VCAT) is a crucial milestone on your journey to veterinary school. It's designed to give you a comprehensive strategy for success, offering guidance on understanding the exam, creating an effective study plan, and using resources to maximize your preparation.

1. Overview of VCAT

Understand the structure and content of VCAT. The exam usually covers areas such as biology, chemistry, physics, reading comprehension and quantitative reasoning. Familiarize yourself with the format, question types and time constraints to take a focused approach to your preparation.

2. Strategies for successful test preparation

Create a systematic and effective study plan tailored to your strengths and weaknesses. Consider your preferred learning style; whether it's visual, auditory, or hands-on and incorporate a variety of study methods, including practice tests, flashcards, and group discussions.

Set a realistic timeline leading up to the exam date.

3. Study resources and tips

Explore a range of resources to enhance your VCAT preparation. Use official study guides, practice exams, and review materials provided by testing agencies. Look for reputable online platforms, review books and interactive tools designed specifically for VCAT preparation. Attend workshops or join study groups and benefit from collaborative learning.

4. Diagnostic Testing and Self-Assessment

Take diagnostic tests to identify your strengths and areas that need improvement. Regular self-assessment will help you monitor your progress and adjust your study plan accordingly. Focus on improving your test-taking strategies, time management skills, and content mastery as the exam date approaches.

5. Time management techniques

The VCAT is a timed exam and effective time management is essential. Practice time-conscious approaches to each section and develop strategies to allocate your time wisely. Find out which question types take more or less time to ensure you can complete the entire exam within the allotted time frame.

6. Test execution strategy

Develop effective test-taking strategies to navigate a variety of question formats. Learn how to prioritize questions, manage stress during the exam and guess correctly when needed. Improve your ability to interpret and analyze information quickly and accurately.

7. Addressing Weaknesses and Seeking Help

If you discover specific weaknesses during preparation,

address them immediately. Seek
help from professors, tutors, or
online resources to clarify
concepts you find challenging.
Work together with coworkers to
obtain a variety of viewpoints and
insights.

8. Balancing VCAT preparation
with other responsibilities

Maintain a healthy balance
between VCAT preparation and
other responsibilities. Prioritize
self-care, getting enough sleep,
and managing stress. Create a
study routine that aligns with
your overall well-being, allowing
you to approach the exam with
confidence and focus.

9. Simulation of test conditions

Simulate exam conditions during practice to familiarize yourself with the testing environment. Simulate actual exam timing and conditions to build confidence and reduce test day anxiety.

10. Reflection and adjustment

Regularly reflect on your progress and adjust your study plan as needed. Be flexible in adapting to new challenges or insights gained during the preparation process. Continuous improvement is key to maximizing your VCAT preparation.

Orientation in the Veterinary School Application Process

The veterinary school application process is a pivotal step in your journey to becoming a veterinarian. This provides a comprehensive guide to creating a convincing application, including preparing application materials, understanding selection criteria and strategic orientation in the admissions process.

1. Understanding Veterinary School Admission Requirements

Familiarize yourself with the specific admissions requirements of the veterinary schools you plan to apply to. Requirements can vary, but commonly include academic transcripts, letters of recommendation, personal statements, and standardized test scores. Make sure you meet all prerequisites and deadlines.

2. Creating a strong personal statement

Your personal statement is an opportunity to express your passion for veterinary medicine, showcase your experience and express your aspirations. Create a compelling story that highlights your unique journey, your commitment to the profession, and the qualities that make you a strong candidate.

3. Selecting and securing strong letters of recommendation

Choose recommenders who can provide insight into your academic ability, character, and suitability for veterinary school. Request letters well in advance and give recommenders plenty of time to write thoughtful and tailored recommendations. After receiving their support, follow up with a thank you letter.

4. Presentation of academic excellence

Highlight your academic achievements throughout the application. Emphasize coursework, research experience, and academic honors that demonstrate your dedication to learning and your readiness for the rigorous curriculum of veterinary school.

5. Documenting veterinary and animal experience

Veterinary schools value hands-on experience with animals. Describe your experience in veterinary clinics, research projects, volunteer work or other relevant settings. Show that you understand the profession and its demands, and highlight how these experiences shaped your commitment to becoming a veterinarian.

6. Demonstration of extracurricular involvement and leadership

Emphasize your participation in leadership positions, extracurricular activities, and volunteer work. Show how these experiences have contributed to your personal and professional growth, demonstrate your ability to balance responsibilities and contribute to a collaborative environment.

7. Preparation for interviews

Make sure you are ready for the interview if you are chosen for one. Prepare your responses to frequently asked interview questions in advance. Demonstrate your communication skills, professionalism and passion for veterinary medicine. Research each school's specific interview format and tailor your preparation accordingly.

8. Navigation in the application service of the Faculty of Veterinary Medicine (VMCAS)

Most veterinary schools in the US use the Veterinary Medical

College Application Service (VMCAS). Learn about the VMCAS application process, including creating an account, entering academic information, and submitting required documents. Pay attention to the deadlines and apply well in advance.

9. Tailoring your application to each school

While using VMCAS simplifies the application process, individual veterinary schools may have additional requirements. Tailor your application to each school by addressing specific questions or challenges listed in their supplemental materials. Show your knowledge and enthusiasm for each institution.

10. Understanding Holistic Admissions and Selection Criteria

Many veterinary schools take a holistic approach to an admission that considers not only academic achievement, but also personal qualities, experience and diversity. Understand each school's selection criteria and highlight how your unique qualities align with their mission and values.

Chapter Four

Excelling in Vet School

Congratulations on your acceptance to veterinary school! Now begins an exciting and challenging journey. It serves as your guide to navigating the academic rigor, clinical experiences, and personal growth that define the veterinary school experience.

1. Acceptance of Academic Rigor

Veterinary school requires rigorous academic commitment. Establish productive study habits, time-management techniques, and organizing principles. Be actively involved in lectures, labs and clinical rotations. Look for academic support resources offered by the school, such as tutoring and study groups.

2. Development of clinical skills

Clinical experience is an integral part of veterinary education. Refine your clinical skills through practical rotations, hands-on sessions and internships. Take advantage of the opportunity to work with different species of animals and improve your diagnostic and treatment skills under the guidance of experienced doctors.

3. Promotion of Professionalism and Ethical Behavior

Maintain a high standard of professionalism and ethical behavior. Adhere to the principles of veterinary ethics and respect the well-being of people and animals. Demonstrate effective communication with colleagues, clients and teachers. Engage in reflective practices to continually improve your professional character.

4. Work-life balance

Veterinary school can be intense and maintaining a healthy work-life balance is essential. Prioritize self-care, adequate sleep, and recreational activities. Create routines that support your well-being, allowing you to maintain energy and enthusiasm throughout the program.

5. Cooperation with colleagues and faculty

Collaborate with your peers and build strong relationships with faculty members. Veterinary medicine is a collaborative field and the support of your colleagues and mentors is invaluable. Join study groups, engage in discussions and seek advice from an experienced teacher.

6. Conducting research and specializations

Explore opportunities for research and specialization in veterinary medicine. Get involved in research projects that align with your interests. Consider taking electives or other certifications in specialized areas to expand your knowledge and skills within the profession.

7. Networking and building a professional identity

Attend conferences, workshops and networking events within the veterinary community. Build connections with professionals, potential mentors and future colleagues. Cultivate your professional identity by actively participating in veterinary organizations and staying informed about developments in the field.

8. Review of Clinical Rotations and Internships

Clinical rotations and internships offer immersive experiences in veterinary practice. Approach these opportunities with enthusiasm and a willingness to learn. Seek feedback from teachers, ask questions, and actively engage in patient care. Use these experiences to enhance your clinical judgment and decision-making skills.

9. Finding Support and Resources

If you encounter problems, seek support from available resources. Many veterinary schools offer counseling services, mentoring programs, and academic assistance. Don't hesitate to reach out to teachers, counselors or classmates for advice and support.

10. Future Planning

As you progress through veterinary school, consider your future career goals. Explore different veterinary specialties, industries and practice settings. Seek mentorship from experienced professionals who can provide insight into different career paths. Create a plan that aligns with your passions and aspirations.

Gain Practical Experience through Clinical Rotations

Clinical rotations are a core aspect of veterinary education and provide hands-on experiences that combine theoretical knowledge with practical skills. This will walk you through the importance of clinical rotations, how to make the most of these experiences, and the

keys to success in a clinical
setting.

1. Understanding the importance of clinical rotations

Clinical rotations are a bridge between classroom learning and real veterinary practice. These rotations provide opportunities to apply theoretical knowledge, develop clinical skills, and gain exposure to a variety of cases. They play a key role in preparing for the dynamic challenges of veterinary medicine.

2. Navigation in different clinical specialties

During clinical rotations, you will have the opportunity to explore different specialties in veterinary medicine. From small animal medicine and surgery to large animal practice, exotic species and more, each rotation offers a unique learning experience. Embrace a variety of specialties to expand your skills and discover potential areas of interest.

3. Development of clinical skills and diagnostic abilities

Clinical rotations provide a hands-on environment to hone your clinical skills and diagnostic abilities. Be actively involved in patient care under the guidance of experienced physicians, from performing physical examinations and diagnostic tests to interpreting results and formulating treatment plans.

4. Building effective communication with clients

Effective communication is the cornerstone of veterinary practice. Learn to communicate clearly and empathetically with clients, convey complex medical information in an understandable way. Develop skills in discussing treatment options, obtaining informed consent and providing advice on pet care.

5. Adopting a collaborative team approach

Veterinary care is a collaborative effort involving a variety of team members, including veterinarians, veterinary technicians, and support staff. Actively engage in a team approach to patient care on rotations. Learn to collaborate, delegate responsibilities and value the contributions of each team member.

6. Adaptation to a rapidly changing environment

Clinical settings can be fast and dynamic. Adaptability is a key attribute during rotations. Be prepared to handle emergencies, sudden changes in patient status, and a diverse workload. Cultivate resilience and a calm demeanor to meet the challenges of a busy clinical environment.

7. Seeking mentorship and constructive feedback

Take advantage of mentoring opportunities available during clinical rotations. Create relationships with experienced physicians who can guide you, share insights, and provide constructive feedback on your performance. Actively seek opportunities to improve your knowledge and skills based on mentor feedback.

8. Balancing observation with hands-on participation

While observing experienced physicians is essential, actively seek opportunities for hands-on participation. Perform procedures under supervision, engage in patient care activities and take responsibility for certain aspects of cases. Balancing observation with active participation accelerates your learning and skill development.

9. Keeping a reflective diary

Keep a reflective journal to document your experiences, challenges, and lessons learned during your clinical rotations. Regularly review and reflect on your progress, identify areas for improvement and set goals for future rotations. A reflective approach increases your self-awareness and contributes to continuous professional development.

10. Demonstrating Professionalism and Ethical Behavior

In the clinical environment, professionalism is paramount. Adhere to ethical standards, demonstrate integrity and prioritize patient well-being. Respect client confidentiality, maintain a positive attitude and demonstrate a commitment to continuous learning and improvement.

Chapter Five

Thriving In Externships and Internships

Externships and internships are an invaluable part of veterinary education and offer immersive experiences in real veterinary practice. This will guide you through the nuances of these opportunities and provide you with information on how to thrive, make meaningful contributions, and lay the foundation for a successful veterinary career.

1. Recognizing the differences: internships vs. externships

Understanding the differences between externships and

internships is essential.
Externships are typically short-term, voluntary experiences designed to observe and learn. Internships, on the other hand, are longer-term, structured programs with a higher degree of involvement and responsibility.

2. Setting clear learning objectives

Set clear learning goals for your externship or internship. Communicate with your supervisor to define your goals, areas of focus and expectations. A well-defined plan will enhance your learning experience and ensure that you acquire a wide range of skills.

3. Adopting a proactive mindset

Approach externships and internships with a proactive mindset. Demonstrate initiative, a desire to learn and a willingness to take responsibility. Look for opportunities to contribute to the practice, whether it's assisting with procedures, engaging clients, or participating in case discussions.

4. Development of effective communication skills

Effective communication is paramount in veterinary practice.

Improve your communication skills by interacting with clients, colleagues and support staff. Learn to communicate information clearly, empathetically discuss treatment options, and work collaboratively with the veterinary team.

5. Navigation in challenging cases with resilience

Externships and internships expose you to a variety of workloads, including challenging cases. Approach these situations with resilience, seek guidance from experienced mentors, and draw on your training. Learn from

each case, adapt and grow as a
veterinary professional.

6. Building Professional Relationships

Cultivate professional relationships with veterinarians, veterinary technicians, and support staff during your externship or internship. Network with industry professionals, seek mentorship, and actively engage in team dynamics. Building strong relationships fosters a positive and collaborative work environment.

7. Adaptation to Different Practice Settings

Veterinary practice varies widely, from small animal clinics to large animal hospitals and specialty practices. Adaptability is key when transitioning between different practice settings during internships or internships. Learn to navigate different environments and appreciate the nuances of each.

8. Demonstrating ethical and compassionate care

Prioritize ethical and compassionate care in all interactions with animals and clients. Adhere to the highest standards of veterinary ethics and put the well-being of patients first. Demonstrate empathy, integrity and a commitment to providing excellent care.

9. Balancing Workload and Self-Service

The requirements for externships and internships can be intense. Find a balance between workload and self-care. Prioritize adequate rest, nutrition and recreational activities. Realize that it is important to maintain your well-being to maintain your effectiveness in a challenging veterinary environment.

10. Seeking Feedback and Continuous Improvement

Actively seek feedback from supervisors and peers to assess your performance. Use constructive feedback as a tool for continuous improvement. Reflect on your experiences, identify areas of growth, and set goals for continued professional development.

Preparation for Licensing and Certification

As you near the culmination of your veterinary education, preparing for licensure and certification is a critical step toward entering the professional realm. This provides an overview of the licensing process,

certification options, and
strategies to ensure success in
obtaining the necessary
credentials.

1. Understanding License
Requirements

Licensing is a mandatory step for
the practice of veterinary
medicine. Familiarize yourself
with the licensing requirements in
the region or country where you
intend to practice. Requirements
may include completing an
accredited veterinary program,
passing licensing exams, and
meeting other criteria such as
clinical experience.

2. Navigating the License Exam Process

Most regions require passing a licensing exam to practice veterinary medicine. Understand the format and content of the exam, which often includes both national and state components. Create a comprehensive study plan, use study resources and consider taking overview courses to enhance your preparation.

3. Preparation for the North American Veterinary Licensing Examination (NAVLE)

If you are seeking licensure in North America, the North

American Veterinary Licensing Examination (NAVLE) is a key component. Spend focused time preparing for this comprehensive exam, which covers topics such as medical and surgical care of various animal species, diagnostic procedures, and legal and ethical aspects.

4. Examination of Specialized Certifications

In addition to a basic license, consider exploring specialty certifications in areas such as surgery, internal medicine, dentistry, or pathology. Specialized certifications will expand your expertise in specific veterinary fields and can open doors to advanced career opportunities.

5. Involvement in further education

Embrace the philosophy of lifelong learning by engaging in Continuing Education (CE). Stay informed about advances in veterinary medicine, attend conferences and participate in workshops to expand your knowledge and maintain your skills throughout your career.

6. Compliance with State-Specific Requirements

Explore formal education programs, including advanced degrees, certification courses, and specialized training. Look for opportunities that align with your career interests, whether it's a master's degree in a specific veterinary discipline, certification in a specialty area, or course work to improve your clinical skills.

7. Participation in continuing education courses

Continuing Education (CE) courses offer a flexible and affordable route to further education. Attend workshops, seminars and online courses to deepen your knowledge in specific areas of veterinary medicine. Many veterinary associations and institutions offer CE opportunities to satisfy a variety of interests and specialties.

8. Participation in veterinary conferences and workshops

Attend veterinary conferences and workshops to keep up to date with the latest research, advances and best practices in the field. Conferences provide opportunities for networking, exposure to cutting-edge technology, and interaction with experts, enriching your

professional development
experience.

9. Use of online learning
platforms

Explore online education
platforms that offer a wide variety
of courses and resources for
veterinary professionals.
Platforms like VetBloom, VIN
(Veterinary Information Network)
and others provide access to
webinars, interactive modules
and virtual learning experiences
that can be tailored to your
specific learning goals.

10. Seeking Mentorship and
Collaboration

Mentoring is a valuable part of professional development. Seek out mentors who can provide advice, share experiences and offer insight into various aspects of veterinary medicine. Collaborate with colleagues, engage in case discussions, and engage in joint projects to broaden your perspectives.

11. Contributing to Research and Publications

Get involved in research projects and consider contributing to publications within the veterinary community. Participating in research will not only expand your knowledge, but also contribute to the advancement of veterinary science. Share your knowledge through articles, presentations or posters at conferences.

12. Monitoring Board Certification and Specialization

Consider pursuing board certification in a recognized veterinary specialty. A specialization demonstrates a commitment to excellence and expertise in a specific area of veterinary medicine. Board-certified veterinarians often have expanded career opportunities and make significant contributions to the advancement of their field.

13. Involvement in veterinary organizations and leadership roles

Active involvement in veterinary organizations provides opportunities for networking, collaboration and leadership development. Join committees, get involved in community initiatives and consider taking on leadership roles to contribute to the growth and advancement of the veterinary profession.

14. Adopting a growth mindset

Cultivate a growth mindset that accepts challenges, appreciates effort, and sees failures as learning opportunities. Approach your professional development with curiosity and a willingness to discover new ideas. Embrace the idea that continuous learning is a journey rather than a destination.

15. Balancing work and professional development

Maintain a balance between work responsibilities and personal well-being while prioritizing professional development. Set realistic goals, allocate dedicated time for learning, and ensure that your pursuit of continuous professional development enhances rather than detracts

from your overall work-life
balance.

Chapter Six

Balancing Work and Well-Being

Maintaining a healthy work-life balance is critical to continued success and well-being in the veterinary profession. It offers strategies for navigating the demands of a veterinary career while prioritizing your mental, physical, and emotional health.

1. Realizing the importance of work-life balance

Understanding the importance of work-life balance is the first step to creating a fulfilling and sustainable veterinary career. A balanced life contributes to

overall well-being, prevents
burnout and increases your
effectiveness as a veterinary
professional.

2. Establishing Realistic Boundaries

Set clear boundaries between
work and personal life. Define
specific working hours and resist
the temptation to constantly
exceed them. Communicate your
boundaries with colleagues and
clients to foster understanding
and support for your need to
balance work and personal
commitments.

3. Preference for Self-Service
Procedures

Prioritize self-care practices to nurture your physical and mental well-being. Include regular exercise, enough sleep and a healthy diet in your routine. Take part in things that make you happy and calm down, such as hobbies, reading, and spending time with your loved ones.

4. Use of time management strategies

Create efficient time management techniques to maximize your output. Prioritize tasks, delegate when appropriate, and avoid over-committing. Use tools like calendars, to-do lists, and productivity apps to organize your workload and set aside time for self-care.

5. Taking breaks and holidays

Recognize the importance of breaks during the work day. Short breaks can improve focus and prevent burnout. Additionally, plan and take vacations to recharge and disconnect from work responsibilities. Vacation significantly contributes to long-term well-being and overall job satisfaction.

6. Establishment of Support Systems

Build a support system that includes colleagues, friends and family. Cultivate relationships with individuals who understand the demands of the veterinary profession and can provide emotional support. Share experiences, seek advice and be open about challenges you may face.

7. Learning to say no

Saying no is a crucial life skill for preserving work-life balance. Be realistic about your workload and commitments and turn down additional responsibilities if necessary. Prioritize tasks and projects based on their importance and alignment with your professional and personal goals.

8. Seeking Professional Support

If work stress overwhelms you, seek professional support. Consider consulting with a mental health professional or counselor who can provide guidance and coping strategies. Addressing mental health issues is a proactive step to maintaining overall well-being.

9. Engaging in Mindfulness and Stress Reduction Techniques

Include stress-reduction and mindfulness practices in your everyday routine. Practices such as meditation, deep breathing exercises or yoga can help relieve stress and promote mental clarity. Find activities that resonate with you and incorporate them into your regular self-care regimen.

10. Assessment of professional satisfaction

Regularly evaluate your professional satisfaction and alignment with your professional goals. Assess whether your current role meets your expectations and contributes positively to your overall well-being. If necessary, consider adjustments such as changing practice settings, exploring new roles, or obtaining additional certifications.

11. Promoting a positive work environment

Help promote a positive work environment in your practice. Foster open communication, collaboration and a supportive culture. A positive workplace increases job satisfaction and promotes the well-being of individuals and the veterinary team.

12. Personal and Professional Growth Considerations

Reflect regularly on your personal and professional growth. Celebrate successes, embrace challenges and reevaluate your priorities. Regular reflection ensures that your career is aligned with your values and allows for adjustments to maintain a healthy work-life balance.

Changing Animal Health and Welfare

Your role as a veterinarian goes beyond clinical practice. This explores opportunities to achieve a positive impact on animal health and welfare beyond individual cases. These strategies allow you to contribute to animal welfare on a larger scale, from community outreach to advocacy.

1. Participation in community educational programs

Participate in community education programs to raise awareness of responsible pet ownership, preventative care and

common health issues. Offer
workshops, seminars, or online
resources to educate pet owners
and the community at large about
the importance of proper animal
care.

2. Cooperation with animal protection organizations

Work with local animal welfare
organizations to support their
initiatives. Volunteer your time
and expertise to provide
veterinary care for animals in
need, participate in spay/neuter
clinics, or donate to educational
programs to prevent cruelty and
neglect.

3. Enforcement of animal welfare legislation

Become an advocate for animal welfare legislation at the local, regional or national level. Stay informed about proposed laws, join advocacy campaigns, and lend your voice to support regulations that promote the humane treatment of animals and address issues such as animal cruelty.

4. Support of rescue and rehabilitation efforts

Support rescue and rehabilitation efforts for animals in need. Work with rescue organizations to provide veterinary care to rescued animals, assist in rehabilitation and help find suitable homes for animals in need.

5. Involvement in the global reach of veterinary activity

Consider participating in global veterinary outreach programs to address animal health challenges internationally. Join initiatives that provide veterinary care in underserved regions, contribute to disease prevention efforts, and share knowledge with veterinary professionals in different parts of the world.

6. Contributing to animal health research

Contribute to research projects focused on advancing animal health and welfare. Collaborate with research institutions, engage in clinical trials, and share your experiences to contribute valuable insights to the scientific community. Research contributions can lead to improved treatments and preventive measures for various animal diseases.

7. Promoting Responsible Breeding Practices

Advocate for responsible breeding practices to prevent overpopulation and address genetic issues in companion animals. Educate breeders and the public on the importance of ethical breeding, genetic testing, and responsible pet acquisition to ensure the well-being of animals.

8. Addressing Zoonotic Diseases and Public Health

Educate the public about zoonotic diseases—those transmitted between animals and humans. Promote preventive measures, responsible pet ownership, and hygiene practices that mitigate the risk of zoonotic diseases, contributing to both animal and public health.

9. Participating in Disaster Response and Relief Efforts

Be prepared to participate in disaster response and relief efforts. Collaborate with emergency response teams to provide veterinary care during natural disasters or emergencies. Your expertise can be crucial in ensuring the well-being of animals affected by such events.

10. Mentorship and Training of Future Veterinarians

Contribute to the growth of the veterinary profession by serving as a mentor to aspiring veterinarians. Provide guidance, share your experiences, and offer insights into the diverse opportunities within the field. Mentorship plays a vital role in shaping the future of veterinary medicine.

11. Fostering a Culture of Compassion and Ethical Care

Promote a culture of compassion and ethical care within the veterinary community. Encourage colleagues to prioritize the welfare of animals, uphold ethical standards, and engage in practices that prioritize both the physical and emotional well-being of the animals under their care.

12. Embracing Sustainable Practices in Veterinary Medicine

Explore and implement sustainable practices in veterinary medicine. Consider eco-friendly initiatives, reduce waste, and promote sustainable choices in daily operations. Contributing to environmental sustainability aligns with the broader goal of improving the overall health of our planet and its inhabitants.

By actively participating in these initiatives, you can extend your impact beyond individual cases,

contributing to the broader goals
of animal health and welfare. This
serves as a guide to inspire and
empower you to make a positive
difference in the lives of animals
and the communities you serve.